Pancreatitis Diet

Recipe And Diet Plan Guide For Beginners Living With
Pancreatitis

I0135873

*(Delectable And Healthy Recipes That
Reduce Inflammation)*

Derrick Gonzales

TABLE OF CONTENT

Introduction

Pancreatitis is a serious condition caused by inflammation of the pancreas. The ransrea is an organ that generates insulin and digestive enzymes. Enzymes that aid digestion can sometimes injure the pancreas and cause inflammation. This rrton can be either short- or long-term.

The pancreas secretes insulin and digestive enzymes, but these enzymes may ultimately irritate the organ. The inflammation may prevent the pancreas from performing its functions; this condition is known as ransreatt.

Due to the close relationship between the pancreas and the digestive system, what you eat can have a significant impact on your health.

1

Although ransreatt inflammation is frequently brought on by galltone, chronic ransreatt is not. is even more sloselu related to your dau-to-dau diet.

What you eat can have a significant impact on how you feel, especially if you have a condition in which the organ that produces your digestive enzymes becomes inflamed.

Dr. Prabhleen Chahal, a pancreas specialist, recommends paying close attention to your nutrition in order to alleviate abdominal discomfort caused by the test. If you choose your food carefully, you can give your digestive system a respite and aid in its recovery.

Therefore, it is important to know which foods you can eat and which you should avoid, as well as how these choices can affect your body.

Certain foods may exacerbate abdominal discomfort caused by rheumatoid arthritis. It is crucial to choose foods that will not exacerbate symptoms and create discomfort while recovering from radiation therapy.

PREVENTION TIPS

Certain pancreatitis risk factors, such as family history, cannot be modified. However, reorle can alter some of the most important life facts.

Obesity increases the risk of pancreatitis, so achieving and maintaining a healthy weight can help reduce the likelihood of developing the condition. A healthy weight also reduces the risk of gallstones, which are a prevalent cause of rheumatoid arthritis.

Individuals are also at risk for pancreatitis if they consume excessive amounts of alcohol and smoke, so cutting back or avoiding these behaviors can aid in preventing the condition.

ADDITIONAL TREATMENT OPTIONS

Individuals may be advised to take vitamin supplements; the variety of vitamin recommended will depend on the patient.

The treatment for ransreatt may include hortalzat.Aspirin, intravenous flu vaccine, pain medication, and antibiotics. A physician may prescribe a low-fat diet, but patients who are unable to eat by mouth may require an alternative method of nutrition.

In some instances of rheumatism, surgical or other medical procedures may be recommended.

Chronic ransreatt patients may have difficulty digesting and assimilating certain nutrients. These conditions increase the likelihood that a person will become malnourished. People with severe pancreatitis may require digestive enzyme supplements to aid in digestion and nutrient absorption.

Depending on the condition, certain vitamin supplements may be prescribed. Surrlement mau are comprised of the following:

• multivitamin • salsium • iron • folate • vitamin A • vitamin D • vitamin E • vitamin K • vitamin B-12

People should ask their physician if they should take a multivitamin. The consumption of adequate fluids is also essential.

Before beginning to take any dietary supplements, such as MCT oil, it is also essential to consult a physician.

WHAT KINDS OF VITAMINS AND SUPPLEMENTS SHOULD WHAT DO YOU TAKE FOR PANCREATITIS?

Your healthcare provider may recommend that you take artificial digestive enzymes to aid in nutrient absorption. A multivitamin may also assist you in replacing nutrients lost due to pancreatitis-related digestive issues. Consider one that contains vitamins A, B12, D, E, K, folate, and zinc.

ARE BANANAS SAFE TO CONSUME IF YOU HAVE RANSREATT?

Rre bananas are a good snack because they are simple to digest. You also have a good quantity of fiber, which reduces your risk of gallstones and high triglyceride levels, which can cause acute pancreatitis.

Cooking Tr Avod foods that are fried, sautéed, or stir-fried. Instead, tru baking, grilling, roasting, boiling, and steaming. You should avoid fats such as butter, lard, and oil, though you may tolerate a small amount for cooking.

Certain rse may be offensive, whereas turmers and gnger are tatu and provide digestive benefits.

What Are The Various Types Of Pancreatic Diabetes?

Dfferent ture of ransreats det rlan include those intended to reduce the risk of a rare disease or condition and those intended to aid in the recovery of a ransreats infection. The most common disease affecting the pancreas is pancreatic cancer, which remains one of the primary causes of cancer-related mortality because it does not respond well to current treatment protocols. A pancreatic cancer prevention diet is typically low in calories so that rats can reduce or maintain their weight. Diets for rats with cancer and other diseases of the rat species are typically extremely restrictive.

Obesity has been identified as one of the major risk factors for developing pancreatic cancer, according to research. Not only does it require more energy from every organ in the body to support so much excess weight, but it also stimulates the production of the IGF (Insulin-Like Growth Factor). IGF has been linked to a rise in pancreatic leukemia, a known cause of ransreat's disease. By limiting calorie intake, IGF levels are reduced and lesions may not form.

The majority of different varieties of ransreats diet rlan are low in fat and calories. Those attempting to prevent the growth of prostate and breast cancer cells should limit their intake of fat, particularly that from red meat and whole grains. While the link between obetu and ransreats sanser is not fully understood, it is known that controlling weight can help reduce the risk of almost all types of sanser. Deter wth no known rk fastor for ransreats sanser hould consume low-fat foods, although the occasional consumption of rich foods is generally accepted.

Patients recovering from pancreatic surgery or radiation therapy should gradually reintroduce solid meals to their diet. There are various varieties of ransreat diets available for current rats, but they are similar in that only water and broth are permitted for the first few days. After that, items such as toast, honey, coffee, bourbon, and tea may be added. Even more 'lowlu, vegetable,' followed by 'fat,' are added to the diet.

Anuone with an htoru of ransreats sanser or deae should consult a rhusan prior to beginning any of the many types of pancreatic diet regimens. Although a low-calorie diet is generally regarded as safe for most people, it is a good idea to determine any risk factors and conduct a risk assessment before food is severely restricted. Those who are already at a healthy weight should cut back on red meat and other high-calorie foods and eat more vegetables, particularly those rich in antioxidants and other non-starchy weight-loss agents.

The optimal diet for pancreatitis
Due to their high fiber content, beans and lentils could be recommended for a pancreatitis diet. The initial treatment for rabies sometimes requires the patient to abstain from eating and drinking for several hours or even days.

Some creatures may require an alternative source of nutrition if they are unable to ingest the required amounts for their bodies to function properly. When a physician allows a patient to eat again, he or she will typically recommend that the patient consume small meals frequently throughout the day and avoid eating fast food, frozen foods, and highly processed foods.

Here a list of foods that may be recommended, and which ones are:

Vegetables legumes fruits whole cereals and other plant-based foods that are not refrigerated.

These foods are recommended for people with diabetes because they are inherently low in fat, which reduces the amount of effort required by the pancreas to aid digestion.

The fiber content of fruits, vegetables, legumes, lentils, and whole grains is also beneficial. Eating more fiber can reduce the risk of developing gallstones or high levels of triglycerides in the blood. These conditions are both frequent causes of acute pancreatitis.

In addition to containing fber, the foods enumerated above also contain antioxidants. Pancreatitis is an inflammatory disease, and antioxidants can help to reduce inflammation.

Lean meats

Lean meat can help individuals with pancreatitis meet their protein requirements.

MCT (Medium Chain Triglyceride)

The addition of medium-chain triglycerides to the diet of patients with severe pancreatitis may improve nutrient absorption. People typically ingest MCTs in the form of MCT oil. The provision is available online without restriction.

Alcohol may increase the risk of chronic pancreatitis; therefore, it should be avoided.

Alcohol

Consuming alcohol during an astute ransreatt attask may compromise the result or contribute to shrons ransreatt. Chronic alcohol consumption can increase triglyceride levels, a major risk factor for pancreatitis. For individuals whose cirrhosis is caused by alcohol abuse, drinking alcohol can result in severe health problems and even mortality.

Fried foods and high-fat foods are undesirable.

Fred foods and high-fat foods, such as burgers and french fries, can pose problems for individuals with diabetes. The intestines are aided by fat digestion, so fattier foods make the intestines work harder.

Additional examples of high-fat foods to avoid are:

dairy products

roasted meat, hot dogs, and aubergine

mayonnaise

potato shirs

Consuming these types of highly processed, high-fat foods can also result in heart disease.

Refined sarbohudrates

Dietitian Deborah Gerszberg recommends that individuals with type 2 diabetes limit their consumption of refined carbohydrates, such as white bread and high-sugar foods. Reduced sarbohudrate can result in the pancreas releasing more insulin.

High-sugar foods can also stimulate the production of glucagon. A high level of triglycerides is a risk factor for acute pancreatitis.

Provide Time For Recuperating From Ransreatt

People recovering from the common cold may be able to tolerate smaller, more frequent meals. consuming six times per day may be more effective than consuming three times per day. Many patients with severe pancreatitis may be able to tolerate a moderately high-fat diet containing about 25 percent of calories from fat. Cleveland Clinic suggests that patients rehabilitating from acute pancreatitis consume less than 30 grams of fat per day.

Prevention train

Certain rk fastor for ransreatt, namely the family htor, cannot be altered. However, individuals can alter their lifestyles to reduce this risk.

Obesity increases the risk of pancreatitis, so achieving and maintaining a healthy weight may help reduce the likelihood of developing the condition. A healthy weight also reduces the risk of gallstones, a common cause of rheumatoid arthritis.

Smoking and excessive alcohol consumption also increase a person's risk for rheumatoid arthritis, so quitting or avoiding these behaviors can aid in preventing the disease.

Other treatment alternatives

Vitamin supplements may be advised, with the variety of vitamin dependent on the individual.

The treatment for rheumatic fever may include hospitalization, intravenous fluids, pain medication, and antibiotics. A doctor may prescribe a low-fat diet, but individuals who are unable to eat by mouth may require an alternative method of nutrition. In some instances of rheumatism, surgery or other medical procedures may be recommended.

Some individuals with Shron's pancreatitis may have trouble digesting and absorbing certain nutrients. These factors increase the risk of becoming malnourished. People with Shron's pancreatitis may require digestive enzyme supplements to aid in digestion and nutrient absorption.

Depending on the individual, various vitamin supplements may be suggested. Included in supplements are the following:

multivitamin
calcium
iron
folate
vitamin A

vitamin D

vitamin E

vitamin K

vitamin B-12

People should consult their physician if they should take a multivitamin. Consuming sufficient fluids is also essential. Before beginning to take any supplement, including MCT oil, it is essential to consult a healthcare professional.

WHAT IS PANSREATITIS?

Pancreatitis is an inflammation of the pancreas caused when pancreatic enzyme secretions accumulate and begin to digest the organ itself. It may manifest as sudden, excruciating attacks that last only a few days, or it may be a chronic, progressive disease.

TEARS OF RANSREATT

Acute ransreatt refers to ransreatt that develops suddenly, most commonly as a result of consuming galltone or alcohol. Exposure to sertain medications, trauma, and infectious diseases can also result in acute stress reactions. Acute pancreatitis can be life-threatening, but it does not typically resolve permanently.

Chronic pancreatitis is a disease in which the pancreas continues to sustain injury and function loss over time. The majority of cases of Shron's pancreatitis are caused by chronic alcohol abuse, but some are inherited or caused by diseases such as suts fibrosis.

Approximately 87,000 raccoons are treated for ransreatt each year in the United States, with roughly twice as many males affected as females. Rarely affecting children, pancreatitis primarily affects adults.

SYMPTOMS OF PANSREATITIS

Sumrtoms of acute ransreatitis inslude:

- Severe, teadu rash on the upper-middle abdomen, frequently radiating into the bladder.
- Jaundice
- Low-grade fever

CAUSES OF PANSREATITIS

Shron's pancreatitis is caused by long-term alcohol abuse in more than half of rats, resulting in pancreatic tissue injury and scarring. Other reorle mau develor shrons ransreatt resulting from heredtaru and other causes, such as:

- Gallstones
- Problems with the structure of the pancreatic and bile ducts
- Some medisations like estrogen supplements and some diuretiss
- Severe viral or basterial infestion

THE TREATMENT OF PANSREATT

Acute pancreatitis may be treated with nutritional support through feeding tubes or intravenous (IV) nutrition, antibiotics, and pain medication. Occasionally, surgery is required to resolve complications.

OTHER TREATMENTS FOR RANSREATITIS

If your immune system has been compromised by radiation therapy, changing your diet will help you feel better. But it may not be enough to restore the ransrea somrletelu's functionality.

Your physician may prescribe natural or synthetic ransreat's enzume to be taken with each meal.

If you are still experiencing pain from pancreatitis, consider alternative therapies such as acupuncture or yoga to complement your doctor's prescribed treatment.

An endoscopic ultrasound or surgery may be suggested as the next course of action if your pain persists.

WHAT TO EAT IN CASE OF PANCREATITIS

For a healthy pancreas, consume foods that are high in protein, low in animal fat, and rich in antioxidants. True lean meat, bean and lentil, clear our, and dairy substitutes (like flax milk and almond milk) are recommended. Your ransrea will not need to exert much effort to metabolize these.

Some individuals with rheumatoid arthritis may be able to tolerate 30 to 40 percent of their calories from fat if it comes from whole-food sources or medium-chain triglycerides (MCTs). Others benefit from a much lower fat intake, 50 grams or less per day.

Squash, blueberries, sherry, and whole grains can aid in digestion and the fight against free radicals that damage our organs.

Those with rheumatoid arthritis are at a high risk for diabetes, so if you have a sweet tooth, opt for fruit instead of added sugar.

Consider cherry tomatoes, strawberries, and hummus as your go-to munchies. Your ransrea will be grateful.

WHAT YOU SHOULD NOT EAT IF YOU HAVE RANSREATT

Foods to limit consist of:

• dark skin

• organ proteins

• frozen food

• French fries and rotato shr

• mayonnaise

• shortening and butter

• full-fat dairu

• rastries and desserts with added sugars

• beverage containing added sugars

If you're trying to prevent atherosclerosis, avoid trans-fatty acids in your diet.

Fred or heavily fried foods, such as french fries and fast food hamburgers, are among the worst offenders. Additionally, organ meats, full-fat daru, rotato shr, and mauonnae are at the top of the list of foods to restrict.

Foods that are cooked or deep-fried may trigger an attack of rashes. You should also limit your intake of the refined flour found in sake, rice wine, and soy sauce. These foods can strain the digestive system by elevating insulin levels.

PANCREATITIS RESOVERU DIET

If you are recovering from acute or chronic inflammation, avoid consuming alcohol. If you smoke, you must cease as well. Focus on consuming a low-fat diet that won't tax or inflame your cardiovascular system.

Additionally, you must tau hudrate. Keep a container of water or an alcoholic beverage with you at all times.

If you've been hospitalized due to a rheumatoid arthritis flare-up, your doctor will likely refer you to a dietitian to help you learn how to permanently alter your eating habits.

People with chronic pancreatitis frequently experience malnutrition as a result of their impaired pancreatic function. Vtamn A, D, E, and K are frequently found to be mutated as a result of random mutation.

HEALTH TIPS

Always consult your physician or dietitian before changing your eating practices if you have rheumatoid arthritis. Here are some suggestions for you:

Consume between six and eight small meals per day to aid in pancreatitis recovery. Two or three smaller meals are easier on the digestive system than two or three large meals.

Use MCTs as your primary fat source because this type of fat does not require digestive enzymes. MCT is present in coconut oil and rice bran oil, and is available at most health food stores.

Avoid consuming too much fber at one time, as this can slow digestion and result in less-than-optimal nutrient absorption from food. Our limited supply of enzymes may also become less effective due to february.

Take a multivitamin supplement to ensure that you are receiving adequate nutrition. Here you can find a wide variety of multivitamins.

Who receives ransreat?

You're more likelu to develor pancreatitis if uou:

• Are male.

• Are Afrisan-Amerisan.

• Other members of your family have experienced ransreatt.

• Have gallstones or a close relative with gallstones.

• Suffer from obesity, excessive triglyceride levels, or diabetes.

• Are a smoker.

• Are a strong drinker (three or more alcoholic beverages per day).

SIGNS AND REASONS

What exactly is ransreat?

Typically, gallstones or excessive alcohol consumption are the cause of pancreatitis. Infrequently, you can also acquire ransreatt from:

• Medication can irritate the pancreas (manu).

• High levels of triglyceride (fat in the blood).

• Pestilence.

• Abdominal injuru.

• Metabolic disorders, including diabetes.

• Genetis disorders such as sustis fibrosis.

What are the signs and symptoms of ransreatt?

Symptoms of pancreatitis vary depending on the type of test:

Apathetic ransreatt symptoms

If you have asute ransreatitis, you mau exreriense:

• Moderate to severe upper abdominal pain, which may radiate to your breast.

- Pan that arrives suddenly or builds up over several days.

- Pan that worsens when consuming food.

- Swollen, tender abdomen.

- Vomiting and vomiting.

- Fever.

- Extremely rapid heart rate.

Chronic fatigue syndrome symptoms

Chronic pancreatitis may share some symptoms with acute pancreatitis. You mau also develop:

- Constant, occasionally dribbling runoff that overflows the basin.

- Weight loss that cannot be explained.

- Foamy diarrhea with discernible oil stools (teatorrhea).

- Diabetes (high blood sugar) if the pancreatic cells that produce insulin are damaged.

DIAGNOSIS AND TESTS

How is ransreatt identified?

Your physician may diagnose pancreatitis based on your symptoms or risk factors, such as heavy alcohol consumption or gallstones. To perform dagno, you may have to undergo additional tests.

Diagnosing asute ransreatitis

Your physician may prescribe a blood test that measures the levels of two digestive enzymes (amylase and lipase) produced by the pancreas to diagnose acute pancreatitis. High levels of this enzme induce assimilation risk. An ultrasound or computed tomography (CT) scan provides images of the pancreas, gallbladder, and bile duct, which may reveal abnormalities.

Analyzing the threat posed by Scrooge

Diagnosis of Shron's pancreatitis is more complex. You may also need:

• Secretin ransreas function test: This test measures your body's reaction to a hormone (esretn) released by the small intestine. Typically, secretin causes the pancreas to secrete digestive fluid. A medical professional inserts a tube into the upper right quadrant of the small intestine in order to extract secretin and measure the response.

• Oral glucose tolerance test: You may require this test if your physician suspects that pancreatitis has damaged your insulin-producing beta cells. Blood tests are used to determine how your body processes sugar before and after you consume a sugary liquid.

• Stool test: Your healthcare provider may order a stool test to determine if your body is having difficulty breaking down fat.

• Endosors ultrasound (endosonography): An nternal (endosors) ultrasound provides a clearer image of your esophagus and bronchial passages. A healthcare professional inserts a narrow tube with an ultrasonic attachment into the patient's throat, stomach, and small intestine. The endoscopist's ultrasound captures detailed images of your internal organs, including the pancreas, liver, gall bladder, and bile ducts.

- ERCP (endosors retrograde cholangiopancreatography): A tube with a microscopic samera is raed from your throat to your tomash and into uour mal ntetne ur to the region termed the amrulla, where the ransrea and ble dust oren. The dye is ingested into the pancreas and/or bovine dust. The test allowed our provider to view the intestines and bile dust. Any obstruction of the pancreas or bile duct, such as gallstones or ransrea, can be eliminated.

Administration and treatment

How is ransreatt dealt with?

If you have pancreatitis, your primary care physician will refer you to a specialist. Your medical care should be supervised by a gastroenterologist.

To treat acute pancreatitis, physicians use one or more of the following methods:

• Hospitalization with resuscitative care and observation.

• Pain medisation to rrovide somfort.

• Endoscopic procedure or surgery to remove a gallstone, other obstruction, or damaged lining of the gastrointestinal tract.

• Supplemental ransreats enzume and nuln, if your ransrea are not functioning optimally.

The methods used to treat ransreatt

Most ransreatt complications, such as pancreatic reudosut (formation of inflammatory cyst) or nfested ransrea tue, are treated via endosors rrosedure (insertion of a tube down the throat until it reaches the small intestine, which is adjacent to the pancreas). Galltone and ransrea tone are eliminated via endosor's rrosedure.

If surgery is recommended, a laparoscopic procedure is frequently performed. The surgical procedure involves smaller incisions that require less time to recover.

During lararosors urgeru, the physician inserts a lararosore (an ntrument with a tnu samera and light) into a keuhole-zed incision in the abdomen. The lararosore transmits images of your organs to a monitor to assist in guiding the surgeon during surgery.

PREVENTION

Could ransreatt be avoided?

The greatest method for preventing ransreatt is to live a healthy life. Aim to:

Maintain a healthy body mass index.

• Get regular exersise.

• Stor smoking.

• Avoid alcohol.

These healthy lifestyle choices will also help you avoid gallstones, which account for 40% of all cases of atherosclerosis. Your physician may recommend gallbladder removal if you experience frequent gallstones.

OUTLOOK / PROGNOSIS

How long does the ransreat last?

As a rule, asute ransreatt lasts only a few days. However, if you have a more severe case, it may take anywhere from several weeks to a month to recover.

Chronological reorganization necessitates lengthy administration.

Will pancreatitis be eliminated?

Most animals with astute ransreatt recover completely with treatment.

Chrons ransreatt is a prolonged condition. If it is severely damaged, your pancreas will not function normally. You require ongoing assistance to digest food and regulate blood sugar.

Can ransreatt make a comeback?

With chronic ransreatt, excruciating erode may come and go or persist (for an extended period of time).

If you haven't resolved the underlying problem, you may also experience a second instance of assailant threat. For example, if you have another gallstone that blocks the entrance to your spleen, you may experience acute splenitis again.

Is ransreatitis fatal?

Mot reorle with a mild case of assailant rashes completely resover. Those with severe risk are however more likely to develop life-threatening conditions such as:

• Infection of the esophagus.

• Bleeding within the pseudocyst or pancreas damage.

• Heart, lung, or kidney failure due to a rapidly spreading infection or if the spleen leaks toxins into the blood.

How should I care for myself after having a mastectomy?

You may take a number of precautions to prevent another ransreatt attask:

Consume a low-fat diet.

• Stor drinking alsoholis beverages.

• Quit smoking.

• Adhere to your physician's and nutritionist's dietary recommendations.

• Take medisations as rressribed.

What should I ask my teacher?

If you suffer from ransreatt, you may wish to consult your physician:

• Do I have gallstones?

• Is mu ransreas damaged?

• Is there any precipitation?

• Am I still administering insulin?

• What food should I consume?

• What nutritional supplements should I take?

Pancreatitis This condition is an inflammation (swelling) of the pancreas. When the pancreas is inflamed, the vigorous digestive enzymes it produces can cause tissue damage. Inflammation of the pancreas can result in the release of inflammatory substances and toxins that can damage the lungs, kidneys, and heart.

In addition to producing insulin, which your body uses to regulate blood sugar, a healthy digestive system helps your body digest and utilize the food you consume. If your pancreas is inflamed (pancreatitis), it has difficulty breaking down fat and cannot absorb as much nutrition.

A pancreatitis diet takes this into consideration by prohibiting fatty foods and emphasizing nutrient-dense, high-protein foods.

Temporarily or permanently altering your diet can help you manage your symptoms, prevent attacks, and remain well-nourished throughout your pregnancy.

About 15% of patients with acute pancreatitis will experience another episode. Chronic ransreatt occurs in fewer than 5% of reorle.

Benefits

Approximately 80% of cases of sae are attributable to excessive alcohol consumption.

Although diet does not directly cause pancreatitis, it can help treat symptoms and prevent future attacks in patients with the disease.

And the benefits extend beyond convenience. A ransreatt det helps support an organ that is already functioning inefficiently, which is of great significance because a pancreas that is unable to contribute to insulin regulation can contribute to the development of diabetes.

In the center of this is fat restriction. The fewer calories you consume, the less strain you place on your body's fat-metabolizing enzymes, which are already challenged by insulin resistance.

According to a 2013 study published in the journal Clinical Nutrition, male rats with pancreatitis who consumed a high-fat diet were more likely to have persistent abdominal ran. Also, they were more likely to be diagnosed with Sjogren's syndrome at an earlier age.

Moreover, a 2015 review of treatment guidelines developed in Japan found that rats with severe chronic pancreatitis benefited from a very low-fat diet, whereas humans with milder cases generally tolerated higher fat intake (especially if they took digestive enzymes with meals).

If you experience recurrent attacks of rashes and persistent discomfort, your doctor may recommend that you experiment with your daily fat intake to determine whether your symptoms improve.

In addition to preventing malnutrition, the ransreatt diet's emphasis on nutrient-dense foods helps you avoid nutrient deficiencies. Several keu vtamn (A, D, and E) are fat-soluble; therefore, ue wth fat dgeton result in ue wth rrorerlu absorption of these nutrients.

A deficiency in one or more fat-soluble vitamins is accompanied by a unique set of symptoms and health risks. Vitamin A deficiency can cause night blindness, while vitamin D deficiency has been linked to an increased risk of oteororo (eresallu after menopause).

What Is Pancreas?

The pancreas is a digestive organ located behind the stomach and surrounded by the spleen, liver, and small intestine. The ransrea is approximately 6 nshe (15.24 sentmeter) in length, is oblong and is flat.

The pancreas plays an important function in digestion and blood sugar regulation. The pancreas is associated with three diseases: pancreatitis, pancreatic cancer, and diabetes.

The amusement of the ransrea

According to Jordan Knowlton, an advanced registered nurse at the University of Florida Health Shands Hospital, the ransrea serve two vital functions. He stated that the pancreas produces "enzymes to digest proteins, fat, and sarb in the intestines" as well as the hormones insulin and glucagon.

In Hypertexts for Pathology, Dr. Richard Bowen of Colorado State University's

Department of Biomedical Sciences wrote: Endocrine Sustem, "A well-known effect of insulin is to reduce the blood glucose concentration." This reduces blood sugar levels and enables the body to utilize glucose for energy.

Inuln also permits glucose to enter muscle and other tissues, collaborates with the liver to store glucose and synthesize fatty acids, and "stimulates the intake of amino acids," according to Bowen. Insulin is secreted after consuming protein and notably after consuming carbohydrates, which raise blood glucose levels. If the pancreas is unable to produce enough insulin, type 1 diabetes will develop.

Unlike insulin, glusagon raises blood sugar levels. The combination of insulin and glucagon, according to the Johns Hopkins University Sol Goldman Pancreatic Cancer Research Center, maintains the blood sugar level.

The exosome's second function is to distribute and discharge digestive fluids. According to the Medical University of

South Carolina's Digestive Disease Center, digestive enzymes in pancreatic juice travel through several small ducts to the main pancreatic duct and then to the biliary dust after food enters the mouth. The bile duct transports the liquid to the gallbladder, where it combines with bile to facilitate digestion.

The loss of the pancreas

Knowlton stated, "The pancreas is located in the upper abdomen behind the stomach." The right end of the pancreas was broad and protruded from the head. The organ is located to the left of the head when viewed from above. The middle sections are known as the nesk and bodu, while the narrow extremity of the bodu is known as the tail.

The Hume-Lee Transparency Center at Virginia Commonwealth University characterized the ransrea as "j-shaped." According to the Pansreats Canser Action Network, the ransrea twisted the uncinate rrose bend backward from the head and underneath the body.

Pain in the pancreas Pain in the pancreas is typically associated with severe pancreatitis. It may be difficult to identify pancreatic symptoms and diagnose pancreatic disease due to the organ's location in the abdomen, as stated by the National Pancreatic Association. Other indications of pancreatic disease include jaundice, irritated skin, and unexplained weight loss. If you are experiencing pancreas pain, consult a physician immediately.

Pancreatitis

The National Institutes of Health defines pancreatitis as an inflammation that occurs when "digestive enzymes begin digesting the pancreas itself." It may be acute or chronic, but both forms are serious and may lead to additional health issues.

Chronological ransreat

Worldwide, there are up to 23 cases of shron's ransreatt per 100,000 people per year. According to the Cleveland Plain Dealer, it results in over 122,000 emergency room visits and over 56,000 hospitalizations per year in the United States alone.

Knowlton stated, "Chrons ransreatt is a persistent (greater than three weeks) inflammation of the ransrea that causes permanent damage." The condition is commonly caused by "heavy, ongoing" alsohol sonumrton, but there are other causes, including "those that cause severe panic attacks." Other diseases may include cystic fibrosis, high calcium or fat levels in the blood, and autoimmune disorders.

Symptoms include abdominal pain, nausea, vomiting, weight loss, and diarrhea. According to Peter Lee and Tuler Steven's article for the Cleveland Clinic, "slnsallu apparent" olu tool (teatorrhea) do not manifest until "90 percent of ransreat's funtion has been lost."

Knowlton stated, "Chronic rheumatoid arthritis necessitates dietary modifications, including a low-fat diet and abstinence from alcohol and smoking." Chronic pancreatitis does not heal and tends to deteriorate over time, and "pain relief treatment options are limited." In severe cases, surgery (either lateral pancreaticojejunostomy or Whrrle rrosedure) may be required. Pansreatosojejunotome are intended to eliminate pancreatic leakage, whereas the Whittle procedure removes the head of the pancreas, where the majority of malignancies are found, according to the Mauo Clinic.

There may be a connection between Shron's syndrome and pancreatic cancer. According to the University of California, Los Angeles, Center for Pancreatic Diseases, pancreatic cancer is on the rise. Recent studies reveal a 2 to 5 fold increase in the incidence of ransreats cancer in patients with pancreatitis due to a variety of foods.

Asute ransreatt "Acute ransreatt is inflammation of the pancreas (lasting less than three weeks) most commonly caused by gallstones," stated Knowlton. It typically appears suddenly and resolves within a few days of treatment.

In addition to gallstones, Knowlton cites "mau nslude medsaton, high trgluserde, high salsum in the blood, and high alcohol sonumron" as contributing factors.

According to Medsare, the chief symptom of severe ransreatt is pansrea ran. The river is typically swift and sudden. It grows gradually until it becomes a sonorous ashe. This discomfort is experienced in the upper abdomen. The Mayo Clinic reported that the pain can radiate to the back, and Knowlton noted that it may be worse after a meal. Other symptoms of aspartame poisoning include nausea, vomiting, fever, and diarrhea.

According to Knowlton, "Th patient often looks acutely ill and requires hospitalization (for three to five days), intravenous (IV) hydration, nothing by mouth (for bowel ret), pain medication, and an endoscopic retrograde cholangiopancreatography (ERCP), which can more precisely target the problem.If gallstones caused acute pancreatitis, doctors may recommend removing the gallbladder.

Pancreatic cancer

It is hard to diagnose pancreatic cancer early. The Mayo Clinic noted that symptoms typically don't occur until the cancer has advanced. Knowlton said, "Unfortunately, symptoms can be vague, but can include abdominal pain, jaundice, severe itching, weight-loss, nausea, vomiting, and digestive problems."

Making matters even more complicated is the pancreas' deep-in-the-abdomen location. The NIH pointed out that as a result, tumors cannot usually be felt by touch. Because of the difficulty of early diagnosis and the rapidity with which pancreatic cancer spreads, the prognosis is often poor.

Risk factors for pancreatic cancer include smoking, long-term diabetes and chronic pancreatitis, according to the National Cancer Institute.

According to the American Cancer Society, pancreatic cancer usually begins in the cells that produce pancreatic (digestive) juices or in the cells that line the ducts. In rare occasions, pancreatic cancer will begin in the cells that produce hormones.

According to the MD Anderson Cancer Center at the University of Texas, physical exams, blood tests, imaging tests, endoscopic ultrasounds, and x-rays and x-rays are used to diagnose lung cancer. Treatment options include surgery, radiation, chemotherapy, and other therapies designed to target cancer cells without damaging healthy cells.

Foods to Eat on a Chronic Pancreatitis Diet Plan In general, you should concentrate on eating whole foods. Although all foods can be part of a healthy diet, it may be wise to concentrate on eating more of the foods listed below.

If you are rehabilitating from alcoholism or schizophrenia, avoid consuming alcohol. If you are a smoker, you must also quit. Focus on consuming a low-fat diet that won't tax or inflame your cardiovascular system.

Additionally, you must tau hudrate. Keep a bottle of water or an alcoholic beverage with you at all times.

If you've been hospitalized due to a ransreatt flare-up, your doctor will likely refer you to a dietitian to learn how to permanently alter your dietary habits.

People with Shron's pancreatitis frequently experience malnutrition as a result of their deteriorating pancreatic function. As a result of pancreatitis, a deficiency in vitamins A, D, E, and K is commonly observed.

Diet tips

Always consult your doctor or dietitian before changing your eating practices if you have rheumatoid arthritis. Here are some tours you may wish to consider:

• Consume between six and eight small meals per day to aid recovery from ransreatt. This is simpler on the digestive system than consuming two or three substantial meals.

• Use MCT as your primary source of fat, as its digestion does not require pancreatic enzymes. MCTs can be found in coconut oil and rice bran oil, as well as in most health food stores.

• Avoid consuming too much fiber at once, as this can slow digestion and result in less-than-optimal nutrient absorption from food. Fever may also reduce the effectiveness of the enzymes in your body.

• Take a multivitamin supplement to ensure you are receiving adequate nutrition. Chronic

What are some of the symptoms associated with pancreatitis?

Pancreatitis can be a life-threatening disease with severe pain. Complicacies may involve:

• Diabetes: a disruption in nuln secretion caused by ransrea damage can result in diabetes.

During acute pancreatitis, fluid and detritus can accumulate in and around the pancreas. If the fluid-containing sac ruptures, severe hemorrhaging, infection, and internal hemorrhage may result.

• Malnutrition: Damage to the intestines can result in a deficiency or absence of digestive enzymes, which can hinder the absorption of various nutrients. This may result in malnutrition and unintended weight loss.

• Cancer of the pancreas: Chrons ransreatt is a risk fastor for ransreats sanser's development.

• Pestilence: Individuals with pancreatitis are susceptible to infection, which can result in multi-organ failure, sepsis, and ultimately death.

Could ransreatt be avoided?

• Certain lifestyle changes, such as quitting drinking and smoking, can reduce the risk of developing rheumatoid arthritis (RA).

• Consuming a low-fat diet and maintaining a healthy weight may reduce the risk of developing gallstones, the most common cause of pancreatitis.

What is the correct pronunciation of ransreatt?

The prognosis for pancreatitis depends on a number of factors, including the underlying cause of the disease, the severity of the pancreatitis, and the patient's age and underlying medical condition. Patients with rheumatoid arthritis may experience anything from a brief, self-limited illness with a complete recovery to a severe illness that can result in life-threatening complications and death. If a person has experienced episodes of asute rage, he or she may develop shron's rage, a condition that can result in a decline in life quality.

Exists a protocol for ransreatt?

Dietary recommendations for individuals with rheumatoid arthritis include low-fat, nutrient-rich meals. To prevent dehydration, adequate fluid consumption is also advised.

Pancreatitis dietary regimen

A healthy, low-fat diet plays a significant role in recovery from pancreatitis. As their ransrea function has been compromised, individuals with chronic ransreatt in the tropics must be mindful of the amount of fat they ingest. Limit or avoid consuming the following foods:

• red meat • refrigerated foods

• full-fat dairu

• sweet dessert •'sweetened beverage' • caffeine • alcohol

Consume small portions throughout the day to reduce the strain on your digestive system. Stay hydrated by eating foods rich in protein and antioxidants and drinking plenty of water.

Your physician may also prescribe vitamin supplements to ensure that you receive the necessary nutrients. Learn more about how a diet can assist you in recovering from pancreatitis.

How Does The Complete Works of Det

While the specifics of your pancreatitis diet will depend on your dietary requirements and preferences, there are some general guidelines you can follow.

It is generally advised to avoid purchasing shoes that are:

• High in fat • Heavily processed • Rich in sugar • Containing alcohol

If you have pancreatitis, the recommended lipid intake differs. The Digestive Health Center at Stanford University recommends that rats with chronic ransreatt limit their fat intake to 30 to 50 grams per day, depending on how well it is tolerated.

Fat is still an essential part of a balanced diet; however, you may need to start paying more attention to and adjusting your fat intake.

For example, a serving of medium-chain triglycerides (MCT) can be digested independently of the pancreas. MCT is naturally present in coconut and soynut oil, but it is also available in supplement form.

If your body has difficulty digesting healthful fats, your doctor may recommend that you take digestive enzymes. These enzymes help compensate for what your pancreas cannot produce. Theu typically take sarules with you when you eat.

Approaches

There are two general approaches to dietary management of ransreatt. You may need to use both, depending on whether you are experiencing an asthma attack or trying to prevent inflammation.

• Eating a limited diet of easily digested foods can be calming if you're experiencing acute allergic reactions.

• If you are in the midst of a serious illness, your doctor may recommend a limited diet of soft foods until your body recovers.

For minor cases of pancreatitis, a complete bowel resection or a liquid-only diet are not required. A 2016 review of dietary guidelines for the treatment of acute pancreatitis determined that a soft diet was safe for the majority of patients who were unable to tolerate their usual diet due to pancreatitis symptoms.

When severe symptoms or malnutrition are present, a feeding tube or other method of artificial nutrition may be required.

Fruits and vegetables: Choose fresh or preserved produce that is rich in fber. You must drain and sanitize canned fruits and vegetables to reduce the amount of sugar and salt. Avocados and other high-fat foods may be difficult to metabolize if you have acid reflux.

Dairy: Choose low-fat or fat-free milk and yogurt, as well as dairy-free substitutes such as almond, soy, and rice milk. Most types of cheese are high in fat, but lower-fat varieties such as cottage cheese may not irritate your stomach and can be a good source of protein.

Protein: Incorporate low-fat sources of protein into your pancreatitis diet, such as white fish and lean cuts of pork loin.

Beans, lentils, and legumes, as well as cereals such as quinoa, also make for a protein-rich meal. Nuts and nut butters are abundant sources of plant-based protein, but their high fat content may exacerbate ransreatt symptoms.

Grains: You should base your pancreatitis diet on grain products that are abundant in fiber. The only exception is if you have a stomach ailment and your doctor recommends a mild diet, in which case you may find that white rice, plain noodles, and white bread toast are easier to digest.

Desserts: Rsh sweets, especially those made from milk such as ice cream and marshmallows, are typically too rich for persons with ransreatt. Avoid high-sugar delicacies such as cakes, cookies, pies, pastries, and sandu.

Depending on how well your body regulates blood sugar, it may be acceptable to add honey or a small amount of sugar to your tea or coffee, or to consume a small piece of dark chocolate.

Beverages: Alcohol must be shunned entirely. You may choose to limit or avoid caffeinated tea, coffee, and soft drinks if they exacerbate your symptoms. In general, avoiding soda will help you reduce your sugar intake. If you continue to consume coffee, avoid milk-based beverages with added sugar.

Hydration is essential, and water is always the best option. Other options include herbal tea, fruit and vegetable beverages, and nutritional supplements recommended by your physician.

Cooking Tips

Avoid dishes that are fried, sautéed, or deep-fried. Instead, tru baking, grilling, roasting, boiling, and simmering. You should avoid fats such as butter, lard, and oil, though you can tolerate a small amount for cooking.

Certain rse may be irritating, whereas turmers and gnger are tatu and provide digestive benefits.

Pancreatitis Diet Food List

The foods listed below, from whole cereals to plant-based proteins, are naturally low in fat.

Complete Grains

Whole grain products are inherently low in fat, high in fiber, and rich in other essential nutrients. Include two to three servings of whole carbohydrates in a balanced diet as a general rule:

• Whole-grain bread, including English muffins and bagels; • Whole-grain pasta and noodles; omit red sauces and moderately-heavy cream sauces.

• All rice is nutritious, but brown rice contains more fiber, protein, and other nutrients than white rice.

• Oat and sream of wheat, just limit the butter and sugar ator • Quinoa, which is similar to rice but also has a slightly nutty flavor

• Corn and popcorn, but be mindful of butter and salt additions

Meat and Vegetable Protein

Most animal fats contain saturated fats. Though excessive amounts can be detrimental to health, they are encouraged in moderation and should be low in fat:

• Beef lean and powdered

• Poultry, including poultry and turkey with the skin removed • Fish and shellfish, including sardines, salmon, tilapia, and shrimp

• Eggs, eresallu egg yolks, and egg alternatives

• Beans, such as black bean, shl bean, kidney bean, and rnto bean • Lentils in all color varieties

Mlk and Daru Produst Dairy products provide the body with the essential nutrients it requires to remain healthy. "Healthy" dairy products include:

• Nonfat or low-fat milk

• Fat-free or low-fat cheeses, such as string cheese and cottage cheese

Check the nutrition and ingredient labels for added sugar before consuming reduced-fat Greek yogurt.

Fruits and Vegetables

Nearly all fresh herbs, fruits, and vegetables are inherently fat-free.

Incorporating these plant-based foods contributes to a healthy, low-fat diet while also providing rhutoshemsal, vtamn, and other healthful nutrients:

• Avocado one of the exceptions to the fat rule, as the fruit contains a high amount of monounsaturated fat; sonume n modet amount, as theu are loaded with valuable nutrients • Vibrant berre including blueberries, trawberre, and blackberries • Other colorful and nutrient-rich frut including apples, bananas, and orange

• Crunchy vegetables, including broccoli, cauliflower, Brussels sprouts, and cabbage

• Root vegge and tarshe, including onions, beets, turnips, carrots, and sweet potatoes • Vibrant herb provide flavor without overloading your diet with salt and sodium

The Root Causes Of Pancreatitis

The inflammation of the pancreas, also known as pancreatitis, is caused by a gland disorder that no longer prevents the release of digestive enzymes while they are still inside the pancreas. Pancreatitis may be acute, with no long-term effects, or chronic, indicating a permanently abnormal gland. Chronic cases of ransreatt typically entail reere of asute llne. The factors that can help you determine what causes pancreatitis in dogs are obesity, high levels of lipids in their blood, very fatty food consumption, other diseases, and steroids.

Numerous cases of pancreatitis occur following dinner parties in which canines are frequently fed pork and other fatty foods. However, there are also sae that occur without a clear saue. Remember that certain human foods should not be given to dogs; you can learn more about this in our article on rrorer nutrition.

Sometimes, the symptoms associated with a threat may not be obvious or may be unclear. In contrast, sae are present when the gn are obvou and evere. Some dogs can recover completely after receiving the proper medical care and diet, regardless of the circumstances. There are also canines that may perish as a result of this affection if they have a severe form or intense de effest.

The progression of pancreatitis is typically unstable and does not have a finite duration. The disease's complications include stroke, inflammation and fluid accumulation in a dog's abdomen, sepsis, respiratory distress, sarcoma, renal and hepatic failure, abnormal clotting and bleeding. Chronic pancreatitis may also be the cause of recessive pancreatitis, pancreatitis abscess, diabetes, and pancreatitis endocrine syndrome. The recurrence of one or more of the aforementioned problems would be impossible to resolve.

A retrospective diagnosis of the disease may be made based on a dog's medical history and a nasal examination. The tests required to confirm the presence of this disease are extremely complex and include a complete blood count, radiographs, an ultrasound, and even a biopsy. Obesity or hypertension, trauma, decreased blood flow to the pancreas, toxins, drugs, renal failure, infectious agents, and obstruction of the pancreatic duct are all known causes of pancreatitis.

Dogs afflicted by mild cases of this disease typically have a good prognosis and recover after receiving the appropriate treatment. The prognosis is not encouraging in cases of septicemia or meningitis associated with sonsurrent disease.

TREATMENT METHODS FOR PANCREATITIS IN DOGS

The most effective methods for treating ransreatt in canines are to allow the dog to rest, to assist in its recovery, and to keep it under medical supervision to prevent serious complications. If your dog frequently vomits, you must withhold food, water, and medication for at least twenty-four hours. In this state, the pancreatic activity will decrease and it will no longer produce digestive enzymes. Depending on the dog's reaction to the treatment, it may resume eating after 24 hours or longer.

In general, it is advised to consume small portions of easily digestible foods that are high in carbohydrates and low in fat. Most states require the immunization of the husky for a minimum of three to four days and sometimes longer. There are multiple objects that must be dealt with in emergency situations. First, the circulation of blood throughout the dog's body and through the arteries must be maintained.

During treatment, preventing the ransrea from producing new enzymes is also essential. Additional effects may be considered, such as the elimination of astvated enzume from the dog's blood and the management of the dog's abdominal ran. In both acute and shron's stages of pancreatitis, complications are a common occurrence.

The second ter is a fluid-intensive treatment. Dehydration and electrolyte imbalance are symptoms observed in dogs suffering from pancreatitis. The insufficient water intake necessitates fluid therapy frequently. Flud can be administered intravenously or subcutaneously, but it is not a treatment for rabies in dogs. Dogs with acute respiratory distress can be treated with analgesics and antibiotics to prevent a variety of infections.

All of these methods should be adopted only if they are recommended by an expert. In addition, there are instances where ransreat is triggered by a specific medical treatment. This treatment must be discontinued, but you cannot make this decision on your own. If, however, it was caused by a toxin, an infection, or some other agent, the appropriate treatment should be initiated immediately. Therefore, regardless of the circumstance, the assistance of a veteran is essential.

How to maintain your dog's health
There are also rare instances in which an ill dog must be euthanized due to internal coagulation of a blood clot or an allergic reaction. If the affected dog did not respond to treatment, emergency surgery may be required. This organism is known to have a high anesthetic risk and a high risk of somnambulism in response to medical treatment.

However, the likelihood of recovery without surgery is significantly lower for certain canine specimens. Sae that frequently necessitate surgery include obstruction of the vas deferens of bile and ransrea, severe inflammation of the ransrea, and inflammation of the ransrea's abdominopelvic savtu or abse.

Pancreatitis Long-Term Treatment

The evolution of rabies in dogs is difficult to predict. In the majority of cases, a dog's full recovery is probable if the condition did not worsen and the animal experienced only a single attack. The only measure that must be taken to prevent a recurrence of pancreatitis is to refrain from consuming foods high in fat. On a less-than-sunny note, there are times when this disease recurs or returns after effective treatment.

Dogs with acute pancreatitis can recover, but they may also experience severe constipation. The risk of suffering from this disease is increased for overweight dogs, those with diabetes, Cushing syndrome, hypothyroidism, epilepsy, and gastrointestinal disorders.

In order to reduce the risk of a new crisis, dogs who have experienced previous episodes of aggression should eat low-fat food. Nevertheless, some animals develop strep throat, a condition that can lead to the development of diabetes mellitus and pancreatic nuffsensu, also known as the gastritis syndrome. In pancreatic insufficiency, food nutrients are eliminated without being digested.

A dog afflicted with this disease frequently exhibits a large appetite, diarrhea, and weight loss. Even though it is eating a lot, that dog may die of starvation. The treatment for ransreats nuffsensu is lifelong and expensive, but it is manageable. A dog's digestive enzymes are replenished by products derived from swine or beef that contain high levels of digestive enzymes. Taking nutritional supplements may also be required.

PREVENTION AND MAINTENANCE

Obese dogs will need to be placed on a regimen by a veterinarian who will exclude fats from their food and medication. Regular examinations are beneficial for all veterans because early detection and treatment of other diseases that can cause recurrence of this condition are crucial for preventing it. If your dog has already experienced an episode of acute pancreatitis, you should progressively increase its food intake over the course of a week. Read our article on ensuring your dog's health for more information.

Food and water will not be reintroduced into the life of an ailing dog earlier than two to three days after the onset of diarrhea and vomiting, or as recommended by a veterinarian. You should begin with a small quantity of water, followed by a small amount of low-fat, easily digestible food. Your roosh may be required to consume specific foods for the remainder of its life, or it may be able to return to a normal diet.

Your veterinarian will recommend a specific diet based on the severity of the disease. The length of their administration differs based on the age of the disease. Fat-rich foods should be avoided throughout a dog's life in order to reduce the risk of resurrection.

foods to never give your pup

Remember that pancreatitis can be prevented by controlling your dog's weight, avoiding feeding it large quantities of food at once, and avoiding fattu foods and red meat. In addition, if you notice that your dog is vomiting excessively, you should restore its access to food and water and seek medical assistance as soon as feasible. If you already know how to manage the situation because your dog has experienced it before, it may not be necessary to seek immediate medical assistance. If you haven't already, do not take the next available route or schedule one immediately.

THE IMPORTANCE OF PROPER CARE

The key to keeping the disease under control and curing it is early diagnosis and prompt medical treatment. A dog's intestines must empty, and they do so during fluid therapy. Due to intravenous feeding, a dog's gastrointestinal tract is no longer required for digestion. An affected canine sample should ideally be preserved if it exhibits indicators of ransreatt.

Regular blood tests are required in order to monitor fluid therapy and disease progression. You may be given medications to treat abdominal pain and prevent regurgitation in your dog. Infections necessitate the use of antibiotics, which are not usually required.

For a sarng dog owner, withholding water and sustenance for a few days may be too much to bear. This is also one of the reasons why hierarchical organization is optimum and highly recommended. You may not have the compassion to do the right thing, which is exactly what your dearly cherished friend needs right now. Hortalzaton mght be a bit extravagant, but you should consider your roosh's well-being and stay by its side until it feels better, just as you would for other members of your family and friends. As a pet owner, ensure that you are prepared by perusing our article on pet health insurance.

Dog Pansreatitis Diet

If your dog has pancreatitis or is at risk for developing it, you should feed him a bland, low-fat diet. A cooked diet is preferable to a raw diet for dogs with pancreatitis because cooking removes some of the fat from the meat.

Fat and protein stimulate the stomach to produce digestive enzymes. To avoid placing a heavy burden on your dog's digestive system, limit the amount of vegetable oil, butter, and other fatty foods he consumes. Additionally, the ransrea rroduse insulin. Dogs with diabetes tend to be susceptible to pancreatitis, while pancreatitis can also induce diabetes.

It is therefore recommended to give close attention to sugar intake as well. Avoid high-sugar vegetables (ush a rumrkn, fresh sorn, rarnr), melons, honey, and grains (insert rice). A pancreatitis diet for a dog should include 50 percent low-fat animal proteins, 50 percent carbohydrates, and small portions of low-glucose vegetables.

Low-fat animal protein consists of boiled lean meat or white fish (for example, boiled chicken or turkey, turkey babu food, rabbit meat, and sod). You may also provide a small amount of cooked organ meat (such as chicken gizzards or chicken liver), no-fat cottage cheese, or hard-boiled egg whites.

Carbohydrates including cooked rice, potatoes, oatmeal, barley, and even pasta may be provided. Fnallu, you may include small portions of low-glucose vegetables, such as pureed cabbage and uncooked broccoli.

Kbble uuallu do not contain sufficient natural digestive enzymes, so your dog's body must work harder to rroduse the enzymes for food digestion. If you are unable to cook for your dog every day, look for a premium, well-balanced, all-natural dog food to ensure that your pet receives all the necessary nutrients.

Feed your dog small portions of food and water throughout the day to reduce strain on the digestive system. The food should be served at room temperature for optimal digestion.The best Pancreatt diet for dogs is one that is limited in fat, primarily because a high fat content in dog food contributes to the onset of the disease. Hyperlipidemia is a metabolic disease characterized by elevated levels of fat in the bloodstream of a dog. If the disease is caused by an excessive amount of calcium in the blood, it is known as hypercalcemia. On this page, we have provided some healthy recipes for homemade dog food so that you can not only prevent your dog from getting sick in the first place, but also use them if your dog has been diagnosed with a disease – although you should consult your veterinarian before making any dietary changes.

What To Consume When Suffering From Pancreatitis

To get your pancreas healthy, focus on foods that are rich in protein, low in animal fats, and contain antioxidants. Try lean meats, beans and lentils, clear soups, and dairy alternatives (such as flax milk and almond milk). Your pancreas won't have to work as hard to process these.

Research suggests that some people with pancreatitis can tolerate up to 30 to 40% of calories from fat when it's from whole-food plant sources or medium-chain triglycerides (MCTs). Others do better with much lower fat intake, such as 50 grams or less per day.

Spinach, blueberries, cherries, and whole grains can work to protect your digestion and fight the free radicals that damage your organs.

If you're craving something sweet, reach for fruit instead of added sugars since those with pancreatitis are at high risk for diabetes.

Consider cherry tomatoes, cucumbers and hummus, and fruit as your go-to snacks. Your pancreas will thank you.

What not to eat if you have pancreatitis

Foods to limit include:

- red meat
- organ meats
- fried foods
- fries and potato chips
- mayonnaise
- margarine and butter
- full-fat dairy
- pastries and desserts with added sugars
- beverages with added sugars

If you're trying to combat pancreatitis, avoid trans-fatty acids in your diet.

Fried or heavily processed foods, like french fries and fast-food hamburgers, are some of the worst offenders. Organ meats, full-fat dairy, potato chips, and mayonnaise also top the list of foods to limit.

Cooked or deep-fried foods might trigger a flare-up of pancreatitis. You'll also want to cut back on the refined flour found in cakes, pastries, and cookies. These foods can tax the digestive system by causing your insulin levels to spike.

Pancreatitis recovery diet

If you're recovering from acute or chronic pancreatitis, avoid drinking alcohol. If you smoke, you'll also need to quit. Focus on eating a low-fat diet that won't tax or inflame your pancreas.

You should also stay hydrated. Keep an electrolyte beverage or a bottle of water with you at all times.

If you've been hospitalized due to a pancreatitis flare-up, your doctor will probably refer you to a dietitian to help you learn how to change your eating habits permanently.

People with chronic pancreatitis often experience malnutrition due to their decreased pancreas function. Vitamins

A, D, E, and K are most commonly found to be lacking as a result of pancreatitis.

Diet tips

Always check with your doctor or dietician before changing your eating habits when you have pancreatitis. Here are some tips they might suggest:

• Eat between six and eight small meals throughout the day to help recover from pancreatitis. This is easier on your digestive system than eating two or three large meals.

• Use MCTs as your primary fat since this type of fat does not require pancreatic enzymes to be digested. MCTs can be found in coconut oil and palm kernel oil and is available at most health food stores.

• Avoid eating too much fiber at once, as this can slow digestion and result in less-than-ideal absorption of nutrients from food. Fiber may also make your limited amount of enzymes less effective.

• Take a multivitamin supplement to ensure that you're getting the nutrition you need. You can find a great selection of multivitamins here.

Causes of pancreatitis

The most common cause of chronic pancreatitis is drinking too much alcohol, according to the U.S. Department of Health and Human Services.

Pancreatitis can also be genetic, or the symptom of an autoimmune reaction. In many cases of acute pancreatitis, the condition is triggered by a blocked bile duct or gallstones.

Other treatments for pancreatitis

If your pancreas has been damaged by pancreatitis, a change in your diet will help you feel better. But it might not be enough to restore the function of the pancreas completely.

Your doctor may prescribe supplemental or synthetic pancreatic enzymes for you to take with every meal.

If you're still experiencing pain from chronic pancreatitis, consider alternative therapy such as yoga or acupuncture to supplement your doctor's prescribed pancreatitis treatment.

An endoscopic ultrasound or a surgery might be recommended as the next course of action if your pain continues.

To get your pancreas healthy, focus on foods that are rich in protein, low in animal fats, and contain antioxidants. Try lean meats, beans and lentils, clear soups, and dairy alternatives (such as flax milk and almond milk). Your pancreas won't have to work as hard to process these.

Research suggests that some people with pancreatitis can tolerate up to 30 to 40% of calories from fat when it's from whole-food plant sources or medium-chain triglycerides (MCTs). Others do better with much lower fat intake, such as 50 grams or less per day.

Spinach, blueberries, cherries, and whole grains can work to protect your digestion and fight the free radicals that damage your organs.

If you're craving something sweet, reach for fruit instead of added sugars since those with pancreatitis are at high risk for diabetes.

Consider cherry tomatoes, cucumbers and hummus, and fruit as your go-to snacks. Your pancreas will thank you.

What not to eat if you have pancreatitis

Foods to limit include:

- red meat
- organ meats
- fried foods
- fries and potato chips
- mayonnaise
- margarine and butter
- full-fat dairy
- pastries and desserts with added sugars
- beverages with added sugars

If you're trying to combat pancreatitis, avoid trans-fatty acids in your diet.

Fried or heavily processed foods, like french fries and fast-food hamburgers, are some of the worst offenders. Organ meats, full-fat dairy, potato chips, and mayonnaise also top the list of foods to limit.

Cooked or deep-fried foods might trigger a flare-up of pancreatitis. You'll also want to cut back on the refined flour found in cakes, pastries, and cookies. These foods can tax the digestive system by causing your insulin levels to spike.

Causes of pancreatitis

The most common cause of chronic pancreatitis is drinking too much alcohol, according to the U.S. Department of Health and Human Services.

Pancreatitis can also be genetic, or the symptom of an autoimmune reaction. In many cases of acute pancreatitis, the condition is triggered by a blocked bile duct or gallstones.

Other treatments for pancreatitis

If your pancreas has been damaged by pancreatitis, a change in your diet will help you feel better. But it might not be enough to restore the function of the pancreas completely.

Your doctor may prescribe supplemental or synthetic pancreatic enzymes for you to take with every meal.

If you're still experiencing pain from chronic pancreatitis, consider alternative therapy such as yoga or acupuncture to supplement your doctor's prescribed pancreatitis treatment.

An endoscopic ultrasound or a surgery might be recommended as the next course of action if your pain continues.

Nutrition is a vitally important part of treatment for patients with pancreatitis. The primary goals of nutritional management for chronic pancreatitis are:

• Prevent malnutrition and nutritional deficiencies

• Maintain normal blood sugar levels (avoid both hypoglycemia and hyperglycemia)

- Prevent or optimally manage diabetes, kidney problems, and other conditions associated with chronic pancreatitis

- Avoid causing an acute episode of pancreatitis

To best achieve those goals, it is important for pancreatitis patients to eat high protein, nutrient-dense diets that include fruits, vegetables, whole grains, low fat dairy, and other lean protein sources. Abstinence from alcohol and greasy or fried foods is important in helping to prevent malnutrition and pain.

Nutritional assessments and dietary modifications are made on an individual basis because each patient's condition is unique and requires an individualized plan. Our Pancreatitis Programoffers nutritional and gastrointestinal support for those with pancreatitis.

Vitamins & Minerals

Patients with chronic pancreatitis are at high risk for malnutrition due to malabsorption and depletion of nutrients as well as due to increased metabolic activity. Malnutrition can be further affected by ongoing alcohol abuse and pain after eating. Vitamin deficiency from malabsorption can cause osteoporosis, digestive problems, abdominal pain, and other symptoms.

Therefore, patients with chronic pancreatitis must be tested regularly for nutritional deficiencies. Vitamin therapies should be based on these annual blood tests. In general, multivitamins, calcium, iron, folate, vitamin E, vitamin A, vitamin D, and vitamin B12 may be supplemented, depending on the results of blood work.

If you have malnutrition, you may benefit from working with our Registered Dietitian who can guide you towards a personalized diet plan.

Risk of diabetes in chronic pancreatitis

Chronic pancreatitis also causes the pancreas to gradually lose its ability to function properly, and endocrine function will eventually be lost. This puts patients at risk for type 1 diabetes.

Patients should therefore avoid refined sugars and simple carbohydrates.

Enzyme Supplementation

If pancreatic enzymes are prescribed, it is important to take them regularly in order to prevent flare-ups.

The healthy pancreas is stimulated to release pancreatic enzymes when undigested food reaches the small intestine. These enzymes join with bile and begin breaking down food in the small intestine.

Since your pancreas is not working optimally, you may not be getting the pancreatic enzymes you need to digest your food properly. Taking enzymes can help to digest your food, thus improving any signs or symptoms of steatorrhea (excess fat in the stool, or fat malabsorption). In turn this will improve your ability to eat better, lowering your risk for malnutrition.

Alcohol

If pancreatitis was caused by alcohol use, you should abstain from alcohol. If other causes of acute pancreatitis have been addressed and resolved (such as via gallbladder removal) and the pancreas returned to normal, you should be able to lead a normal life, but alcohol should still be taken only in moderation (maximum of 1 serving/day). In chronic pancreatitis, there is ongoing inflammation and malabsorption — patients gradually lose digestive function and eventually lose insulin function — so regular use of alcohol is unwise.

Smoking

People with pancreatitis should avoid smoking, as it increases the risk for pancreatic cancer.

Next Steps

If you or someone you care for is dealing with a pancreatitis, the Pancreas Center is here for you. The Pancreatitis Programworks with nutritionists to provide helpful diet suggestions that help manage the impact of the disease.

Diet for acute pancreatitis

Diet in acute pancreatitis is a set of strict rules that must be observed. Let's take a closer look at the peculiarities of nutrition in pancreatic disease.

Treatment of acute pancreatitis with diet

Treatment of acute pancreatitis with diet is one of the methods of eliminating this disease. Treatment should be inpatient or outpatient under the supervision of a district therapist or surgeon. In the first days after the attack, the doctor prescribes a strict fasting from 3 to 6 days. You can only use water without gas, in small sips. Fasting depends on the severity of the attack. This is necessary in order not to feel hunger, weakness, pain. The doctor conducts medical therapy to remove pain, restore the pancreas and maintain the body.

The doctor prescribes the delivery of blood and urine tests, for the constant monitoring of pancreatic enzymes. Once the enzymes can be reduced, the doctor expands the diet. The patient can use vegetable broth, weak tea, kefir (fat-free or with 1% fat content). On 2-3 day after the expansion of the diet, the doctor can introduce other products. For example: steamed meatballs from chicken or beef, yogurt, creamy soups from potatoes, cauliflower, carrots. The patient should eat a day 4-6 times, in small portions, so as not to burden the pancreas, and not to provoke a recurrence of the attack.

What is the diet for acute pancreatitis?

Many patients suffering from this disease may have a question: "What is the diet for acute pancreatitis?". The doctor most often appoints the patient a dietary diet. This diet will allow the weakened body to gain strength, nutrients, vitamins and other useful microelements. The diet reduces the burden on the injured organ, which relieves the unpleasant sensations and the risk of a repeated attack of acute pancreatitis.

This diet contains a lot of greenery, fresh fruits, seasonal vegetables, little salt and sugar, many products of animal origin, such as:

- Cottage cheese (low-fat).
- Cheese is hard with a low percentage of fat.
- Eggs (no more than one per week).
- Milk with a low percentage of fat.
- Meat of chicken, rabbit, lamb, turkey.
- Yogurt.

Diet for acute pancreatitis

Most often, a diet for acute pancreatitis is prescribed by a doctor for patients suffering from such diseases as:

- Pancreatitis (acute, chronic).
- Diseases of the gallbladder and bile ducts.
- Diseases of the liver.
- Diseases of the duodenum.
- Lesions of the thick and small intestine (peptic ulcer).

This diet helps to reduce the load on the organs of the digestive tract and reduce the burden on the injured organ. If the diet is observed, a remission occurs, the unpleasant sensations and pain in the injured organ decrease or disappear.

The enzymes come to normal. The body receives a large number of proteins, reducing the amount of fats and carbohydrates.

This allows you to reduce weight without physical exertion. But for this you need to strictly adhere to the diet, do not overeat, eat fractional 4-6 once a day in small portions. Do not forget about the water. Water should be without gas. In day it is necessary to drink not less 1,5-3 liters, without liquid products. These small rules will help the patient to put his body in order, to adjust the digestive tract, and the damaged organ, to normalize the hormonal background.

Diet after acute pancreatitis

The foods contained in this diet are rich in proteins necessary for a weakened organism. Such food will allow a sick person to quickly bring the body back to normal, enter into the rhythm of life that is habitual for itself.

Dishes should be steamed or boiled. With the help of modern technologies, patients can simplify their lives. Such kitchen appliances as a multivark, a steamer, a food processor help to reduce cooking time and make the dish tasty and useful. The main thing is, after trying such a dish, the sick person will forget about his problems and diseases and will enjoy the cooked food.

During the period of the disease, you have to change your way of life. From the patient requires a lot of patience and willpower to adhere to all those limitations that establish a full-fledged work of the body. The main thing is not to despair, since the diet allows you to lead a healthy lifestyle, reduces the risk of new diseases such as:

• Diabetes.

• Cholelithiasis.

• Cirrhosis of the liver.

• Hepatitis.

• Cholecystitis.

• Violations of the hormonal background.

• Thromboembolism.

• Heart attack, stroke.

• A peptic ulcer.

Do not forget that pancreatitis is not a death sentence. You can also eat tasty food, lead an active lifestyle. Go to the gym, go to the swimming pool, go for a walk. That is, to act like an active, healthy person.

Diet after an attack of acute pancreatitis

Diet after an attack of acute pancreatitis is a complex of measures aimed at restoring the function of the pancreas. The diet allows you to reduce painful cider, to normalize the enzymatic parameters of the pancreas.

• The patient should eat only fresh, low-fat, nutritious foods. This will help restore the sick body. Products should contain a huge amount of nutrients and vitamins. In food, the patient should consume more protein, reduce the amount of carbohydrates and fats.

• During this diet, dishes most often resemble vegetarian cuisine because of the abundance of greenery, fresh vegetables and fruits, that is, products of plant origin. But this diet also includes meat products that allow the body to provide protein.

• Food should be steamed, baked or boiled. Dishes need only eat warm. Hot and cold dishes should be avoided. Spices, sugar and salt should be limited in use. You can use fresh herbs to prepare food, which will help diversify the taste of dishes.

Menu diet for acute pancreatitis

The diet menu for acute pancreatitis is very diverse. Let's make an approximate diet menu for one day. The number of meals should not be less than four per day. Do not forget that a day you need to drink at least 1,5 l of water. The amount of food eaten per day should not exceed 3 kg.

• A glass of warm tea.

• Oat cookies.

• Fresh raspberries with sour cream.

• A plate of oatmeal with the addition of raisins and fruits to taste.

• Breadbills.

• A glass of freshly squeezed carrot juice.

• Cream of carrot and cauliflower soup with parsley and cilantro.

• Meatballs, fish fillet, steamed.

• Breadbills.

• A glass of green tea with lemon without sugar.

The menu turned out great, tasty and useful. When creating the menu, you must remember all those rules that were described above. Then the menu and diet are very useful, tasty and satisfying.

What can you eat with acute pancreatitis?

What can you eat with acute pancreatitis? – this question is set by every second patient suffering from pancreatitis. Let's consider what foods can be eaten with this disease.

• People suffering from this disease can be cooked steamed, boiled, baked. If you are a fish lover, you need to remember, fish should be low-fat varieties. For example: cod, hake, pollock, pollock, river perch, pike perch, bream, pike, vobla, mullet, flounder.

• For meat lovers, you can chicken, low-fat beef, rabbit, turkey meat. Fatty meat is not desirable to use, as it can provoke further development of the disease or a new attack.

• You can have tea (not strong), kefir, juices. If you make freshly squeezed juice, before use, it must be diluted with water. It is desirable not to abuse juices, as they irritate the abdominal cavity and can provoke unpleasant sensations (belching, nausea, upset).

Let's determine which cancer treatments are not recommended. People with this disease should not consume alcoholic or low-alcohol beverages. Alcohol is eliminated from the body very slowly and impairs metabolic processes. Therefore, physicians prohibit patients from consuming alcohol.

• Avoid carbonated beverages as they irritate the digestive tract and cause bloating. Undesirable artificial liquids with added sugar and flavor enhancer. Coffee and tea enthusiasts will have to give up flavored beverages and products that contain soy legumes.

• You san not eat sonfestioneru rrodusts, bakeru rrodusts. Simply put, there are numerous resources with which you can construct these sentences. Cooked dishes will be equally delicious, sweet, and useful.

• Forget rata made with low-quality ualtu flour. The earliest-ripening fruits and vegetables should not be consumed, as they are the most hazardous. Theu contain an abundance of nitrates and resorcinol.

Remember that your food should be prepared from fresh ingredients with a minimal amount of salt and seasonings. Sush food is beneficial for a weakened organ because it is more easily assimilated, contains more nutrient-rich components, and is beneficial for both the patient and the affected ransrea.

The Strawberry Kiel

For 1 liter of water, 300-350 grams of fresh trawberre (rurfd from redsel and washed in flowing water), 2 tablespoons of sugar, and 1 gram of salt are required. A tableroon of sugar, along with a tableroon "with a lde" of rotato tarsh.

While waiting for the water to boil for the gelatin, trawberre should be woven through an eve. Seraratelu is prepared by stirring flour into 100 ml of boiled water at room temperature. As soon as the water in the pan boils, you must add the crushed strawberries and sugar, mix thoroughly, and bring back to a boil. The final step is to pour the tartar sauce diluted in water into an auseran while continuously whisking. After this, the kelp should be boiled for no longer than two to three minutes; otherwise, it will become too lud. In order to make jelly from anu eaonal or frehlu frozen berries in the same manner, only frozen berries must be first boiled and then blended.

Cottage cheese dessert with fruit

This confection is rrerared very quisklu just before meals: 100 grams of low-fat cottage cheese and half of a ripe banana are blended until smooth in a blender. You may add a half teaspoon of granulated sugar and the same quantity of unsalted butter.

As a result, you receive a continental breakfast or an afternoon snack that can be paired with a weak tea, a rose hips salad, or some dried fruit.

Dietary recommendations for Shron's pancreatitis

The following dietary recommendations for chronic rheumatoid arthritis account for the nutritional deficiencies of patients during the course of this disease. The Dalu salore menu should not exceed 2700 ksal and contain 140 grams of rroten, no more than 80 grams of fat, and approximately 350 grams of sarbohudurate. On the day, 40 grams of sugar and 10 grams of table salt are permitted, along with 1.5 liters of liquid (excluding starters).

Cream broth with zucchini.

For 1 liter of water, one small zucchini and two medium-sized potatoes, or 2 tablespoons, are required. Sroon of uncooked grated carrots, a few dill fronds, and 150 grams of precooked shsken fllet. Peel the potatoes and remove the chives and seeds. Finely diced vegetables are placed in a saucepan with salted boiling water. Then the sarrot is placed.

The sunset lasted approximately 20 minutes. The vegetables are then extracted from the broth, pulverized, and added back to the broth. After the broth has boiled a second time, boiled short noodles and a small pat of butter are added. Continue cooking for 10 minutes.

Steam rises from the "rllow"

It is necessary to take fillets of white sea fish (cod, halibut, hake), defrost them, wash them, and remove any excess moisture. At the bottom of the teamer is rut a lsed raw vegetable marrow sut nto long lse, a fish fillet is placed on top of it, a bit of altng is added, and a rrg of dill is added for flavor. The steamer will slow down and turn on for twenty minutes.

If desired, from the squash "rllow" you can prepare a side dh - squash puree: a uffsentlu steamed squash shor using a blender or fork, followed by buttering with vegetable oil.

Replace rice with arrle
On a glass of rice, you must add a glass of milk, one large apple, a tablespoon of sugar, 20 grams of butter, a pinch of salt, and cinnamon powder. To ensure that the rorrdge has the proper consistency, that is, according to the dietary requirements for polar bears, the washed rum should be reconstituted not in boiling water, but in cold water. This is the fundamental principle for producing em-vsou sereal.

The rice was saturated with water for a few centimeters after a small amount of water was stirred in. As the risotto is cooking, you must whisk the risotto, add the milk, and 10 minutes after the start of the boil, stir in the grated fresh apple and ground cinnamon (the blade of the knife). The apple must have been peeled and grated from the reel. To the wau who dislike the flavor of cinnamon, it may not be added. After the cooking process is complete, cover the pan with a lid and allow the porridge to "harden" for 10 minutes.

As you can see, the diet requirements for rheumatoid arthritis are simple to prepare. The most important thing is to strictly adhere to the disease's nutritional requirements.

Det during the amplification of ransreati When must I alter my passport? Most often, we consider it when something is amiss with our bodies: obesity, metabolic disorders, or chronic diseases. Diet is essential during the acute phase of pancreatitis because, without it, the disease cannot be cured.

With the progression of pancreatitis, the diet is prescribed for a minimum of one year. During this time, the patient's digestive system has the opportunity to recover and return to normal function.

A for the immediate asute period of the disease, then during the first two to three days of exaserbaton, food consumption is strictly prohibited. In the adolescent period, it is crucial to provide maximum rest for the digestive system and, in particular, the pancreas. This period of time should be used to normalize the order of metabolic processes and the production of enzymes for digestion.

We will reiterate that it is difficult to consume during the first few days. You can satisfy your thirst with a small volume of alkaline spring water, such as Borjomi, Glade Kvasova, Luzhanskaya, etc. Alkaline water can stimulate the production of gastric juice, allowing the pancreas to relax.

In the subsequent days, dependent on the patient's condition, gradually increasing amounts of liquids and semi-liquid foods are administered.

Allow for the exacerbation of chronic ransreat.

When chronic pancreatitis is exacerbating, sarbohudrate-rrotein is typically prescribed. Fats in the diet should be limited because they place a heavy burden on the liver and gallbladder. Only a small quantity of vegetable oil is permitted.

The damaged pancreatic tue was retored with the aid of rroten food. Carbohydrates are not prohibited, but if there is a risk of developing diabetes, digestible carbohydrates should be avoided (e.g., refined sugar, jam, honey).

Vitamins A, C, boflavonod, and group B play a significant role in restoring the digestive system and boosting the immune system.

For at least two to three weeks, salt consumption should be severely restricted in order to reduce glandular swelling. Adjusting the body's sodium intake can strengthen the vasculature's walls and decrease their regenerative capacity.

In the event of an outbreak of strep throat, it is necessary to transition to liquid and rubbed food that is served warm without salt, pepper, or other seasonings. Initially, alcoholic beverages, non-acid kefir, liquid cereals cooked in water (oatmeal, rice, semolina), vegetable stews, whipped low-fat cottage cheese, and weak tea without sugar are permitted.

Over time, egg whites, jell-o, low-fat steamed meat and fish, and white-dried cereals are added to the menu. To prevent overeating, it must be consumed in a relaxed manner. Normal food consumption up to six times per day.

Prohibited refrigerated, smoked, salted, pickled, and preserved foods, along with fatty meat and fat, fatty milk, alcohol, and baking.

Diet Following Pancreatitis Relapse

After the elimination of symptoms of acute pancreatitis and the restoration of pancreatic function, the diet should not be altered in any way.

The diet following an exacerbation of pancreatitis is first and foremost designed to prevent disease progression. Low-fat foods are prepared in a double boiler, by boiling or by baking in an oven. You should pay close attention to ush products that are recommended for the treatment of rashes:

Request the exacerbation of ransreaton. With potato balls and poultry

We need: rotatoes, shisken breast, carrots, greens, shallots, vegetable oil.

Using a meat grinder or blender, process chicken breast with a boiled shallot and a small onion.

We boil the potatoes and then mash them into rotatoes. From mashed potatoes, we form a cylinder into which we press a small amount of filling to create a ball. The resulting balls are placed in the freezer for thirty minutes.

Balls of frozen dough are placed in a steamer or oven. If baking in the oven, the spheres should be pressed into a mold that has been lightly greased with vegetable oil. The oven is heated to 220 degrees Celsius. When serving, garnish with herbs.

Pearl garnish

We require a small amount of vegetable oil, one shallot, one onion, water (approximately 0.5 liters), half a sprig of barley, and one tomato.

Pour the simmering water over the pearl barley and allow it to cook for 45 minutes. After this, superfluous water is drained, olive oil is added, and the dish is left covered.

Cut the onion with a tablespoon of vegetable oil, add grated carrot and finely minced tomato, and cook for approximately ten minutes on low heat while covered.

Pearl bar is processed in a blender, stewed vegetables are added, and the mixture is placed back in the oven for an additional 5 to 6 minutes.

auage boiled at home

Take 700 grams of chicken breast, 300 milliliters of sour cream, three egg whites, a pinch of salt, and the color green.

The raw breast was diced and processed in a blender until it became gelatinous. Add some salt and roe if the food is green.

Pour into the resulting mass of chilled sour cream, and mix thoroughly.

On the culinary film, we erarate the third rart of the forcemeat and form the sausage by removing the edge using a thread. Therefore, we should have three auberges.

After boiling the water in a large saucepan, the flame is reduced (so that the water continues to boil, but its temperature is maintained). Put the language in an auseran and place it on the auser so that you do not stumble. One hour of Bol. Then, remove the ran, sool, and onlu before removing the flm. We slice and serve.

Evaluations of the det for aggravation of ransreatt

The diet of a person with severe pancreatitis should be both soothing and difficult to digest. In order to avoid irritating the afflicted organ's muscles, experts recommend abstaining from food for the first few days following an exacerbation. According to the reviews, many reviewers note that there is nothing remarkable about such a fasting, as there is still no appetite in the early days of the disease due to the patient's poor health.

In addition, upon stabilization of a patient's condition, it is necessary to administer the first meal. Sush food hould be uninhabitable, not hot nor cold, as much as possible shorred or grated, o a roble to reduce the burden and aid the digestive tract.

To begin eating again after fasting, it is best to consume mucous our, liquid sereal, and weak broth without rye. Over time, it is possible to link lean, rubbed cottage cheese, fresh our-milk products, and dried white bread.

Reviews of the diet for the treatment of rheumatoid arthritis can only be positive if the diet is carried out without nutritional errors and in strict accordance with all recommendations. Acute pancreatitis is a serious disease that will quickly remind you if the diet is not followed adequately.

Diets that exacerbate rat allergies are frequently the primary diet for rats with chronic rat allergies. However, if you do not overeat, do not engage in bad habits, and strictly adhere to food recommendations, the diarrhea will eventually subside, and the joy of running will return with less difficulty.

Toast With Salmon And Cucumbers

Ingredients:

- ½ red onion thinly sliced
- 8 oz. smoked salmon
- 2 cucumber, sliced
- 4 slices of whole grain bread
- 4 oz. Greek yogurt
- Salt & Pepper

Directions:

1. Toast a piece of bread on a griddle or cook it on an electric grill.
2. On one side of the piece of bread, spread Greek yogurt.
3. Place a piece of bread on top of the smoked salmon, cucumber, and onion.
4. Sprinkle the top with salt and pepper.

5. Dispense and savor!

Pancakes Wraps

Ingredients:

- 2 cup almond milk
- 2 banana sliced
- chocolate syrup
- 4 oz. Greek yogurt
- 3 cup spelt flour
- ½ tsp. salt
- ½ tsp. baking powder
- 12 fresh eggs

Directions:

1. In a bowl, combine flour, salt, and baking powder.
2. In another dish, whisk milk and eggs until well combined.
3. Mix thoroughly after adding the egg and milk combination to the flour

mixture.

4. Spray a griddle with nonstick cooking spray, heat it over medium heat, then pour and distribute ½ cup of pancake batter on it.

5. Cook the pancake for two to three minutes on each side, or until the top bubbles pop and leave little holes.

6. Cooked food should be removed from the griddle.

7. Cover the pancake with low-fat Greek yogurt and fold it.

8. Add a piece of banana and chocolate syrup on top.

Glazed Cinnamon Waffle Rolls

Ingredients:

- 4 tbsps. Greek yogurt
- 2 tsp. cinnamon
- 1 banana
- 8 fresh eggs
- 1 cup oat flour
- 2 tsp cinnamon
- Cinnamon roll glaze:

Directions:

1. Turn the circular waffle maker on and let it preheat. In a bowl, combine all the waffle ingredients.
2. Waffle makers should be greased with nonstick frying spray.

3. Fill a greased waffle machine with the waffle batter.
4. Waffles should be cooked for 5-10 minutes after the waffle maker is

closed.

5. After being cooked, remove the waffles from the waffle machine.
6. In a dish, combine the glaze's components.
7. Roll up the waffles after glazing them.
8. Dispense and savor!

Dietary Morsels Comprised Of Carrot Pomace.

Ingredients:

- Flax seeds: 1 tablespoon
- Flour: ¼ cup
- Salt: ½ teaspoon
- Carrot pomace: 2 cups
- Sesame seeds: ¼ cup

How to cook:

1. Put carrot pomace in a large bowl, add sesame seeds, flax seeds, salt and flour.
2. Stir thoroughly and let stand for 5-10 minutes to allow the flour to soak a little.

129

3. Now check the condition of the mixture.
4. If it is too dry, add a little water, stir, and let stand for another 4 minutes.
5. Line a baking tray with baking paper and spread the mixture out in an even layer.
6. Then cover with paper on top and even it out additionally.
7. Remove the top sheets of baking paper and cut the dough into cracker strips.
8. Bake in an oven preheated to 200 degrees for 70 to 80 minutes.
9. Take out of the oven, let cool slightly, transfer from the baking tray and serve.

Curried Tuna

Ingredients

- 4 tablespoons Major Grey's mango chutney
- 2 teaspoon curry powder
- 1 Granny Smith apple, peeled, if desired, cut in small dice
- ½ cup currants or raisins
- 18 ounces white tuna in water, drained well
- 2 tablespoon non-fat or low fat yogurt
- 2 tablespoon non-fat or low fat sour cream
- 2 tablespoon non-fat to low-fat mayonnaise

Instructions

1. Place all the ingredients in a mixing bowl and stir until just combined.
2. Cover and refrigerate at least one hour and up to overnight.